Oxford Centre for

Healthy Sleep

The Oxford Centre for the Mind:

Quick Courses

Gary Lorrison

Healthy Sleep

The Oxford Centre for the Mind

Quick Courses

Strategies, techniques and advice to ensure that you gain good quality rest and sleep

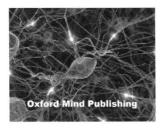

Gary Lorrison

Oxford Mind Publishing

Oxford Centre for the Mind

THE OXFORD CENTRE FOR THE MIND LIMITED

#123,
94, London Road
Headington
Oxford OX3 9FN

email: info@oxfordmind.co.uk
web: www.oxfordmind.co.uk

Oxford Mind Publishing is a division of the Oxford Centre for the Mind Limited.

ISBN-13: 978-1499670141

ISBN-10: 1499670141

About the Author

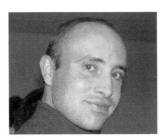

Having studied law at Cambridge, Gary Lorrison started off his career working in London as a solicitor but quickly saw the light and left the legal profession to develop his interest in the mind. He quickly earned two degrees in philosophy but found himself focusing on how one could use the techniques of philosophy, psychology and science to run one's mind more effectively.

Since 2003, he has been actively involved in running personal development training programmes to help people improve their mental performance. He has a special interest in memory training and other ways of helping people absorb information as well as the techniques of logical, critical and analytical thinking and the limits of human rationality.

In his spare time he enjoys walking in the countryside, takes a keen interest in music playing a number of instruments and is an occasional skydiver.

He lives on a farm near Oxford with four dogs, three cats, three ducks, six geese, about five hundred sheep and the occasional human being.

Testimonials

Testimonials for our seminars: -

"Excellent - best course I have been on in ages - thought provoking and insightful"

"Great workshop. Coach created a very relaxing, easy and open atmosphere. Coach was helpful and had a very pleasant way of interacting with us"

"I am very happy I came to this workshop. It was good value for money and provided very useful skills that I know will help my studies"

"It's a great course - I would recommend you go on it"

"Good fun and value for money"

"Do it! - Very interesting and a good approach to de-stressing about work levels etc."

"It really works, especially the visualisation techniques"

For information on all of the courses run by the Oxford Centre for the Mind please visit our website:

www.oxfordmind.co.uk

Healthy Sleep

Contents

Healthy Sleep

ONE

INTRODUCTION

Aim

The aim of this *Sleep Course* is to ensure that you obtain the best quality sleep that you possibly can. If you have read through the other courses within the *Oxford Centre for the Mind* series you will by now be aware that, to perform at optimal levels at all times, you need to be properly rested. The quality of your waking lives is determined by the quality of your sleep and so to function at optimal levels throughout your life, it is vital that you obtain good quality sleep.

Only one in five people are regularly able to get to sleep with little or no effort. The remainder will need some help at certain points during their lives. This course will help you to rest and sleep well.

Benefits

If you improve the quality of your sleep you will notice a number of benefits. These include the following: -

- Obtaining good quality sleep over the long term is one of the easiest ways to ensure that you live a long, healthy life.

- Good sleep will help you to get through the day more efficiently. By being properly rested you will be fully energised and not prone to concentration lapses during the day.

- Higher energy levels throughout the day will ensure that your mind is more focused and your mental powers are enhanced. Moreover, proper rest will give your body time to recover after exercise, ensuring that your physical performance is optimised.

- Obtaining proper rest will mean that you enjoy life more, are less prone to mood swings and increase your chances of living a long and happy life. It may even help you to live longer.

- Good sleep can lead to an improvement in performance of a variety of tasks in different fields both at home and at work. It has been estimated that productivity at work increases by about twenty per cent when workers obtain good quality sleep.

If you follow this course you will: -

- Rid yourself of excessive sleepiness
- Feel more alert
- Get to sleep at night more easily
- Start to sleep well all the way through the night until it gets light
- Reduce your chances of accidents and injuries, including car accidents
- Feel better both physically and psychologically.

Beliefs

Sleep is an integral part of your life. We spend about a third of our lives asleep, which is a very significant proportion, yet most of us devote very little thought to how we sleep. It is important to master sleep if you want to be able to perform at your highest levels throughout your life.

Many people believe that you need to get a full eight hours sleep in order to be fully rested. This is not necessarily true. Your goal should be to obtain enough sleep to be refreshed and alert when you are awake throughout the day. This course will help you to determine how much sleep you need.

People often believe that the quality of their sleep is likely to get worse as they get older. This need not be the case at all if sleep is properly planned. As with most other areas of life, if you start to take care of your sleep now, you will be able to have good refreshing, high quality sleep throughout your life.

If you do not get good sleep, you are likely to suffer from a number of unwelcome symptoms. Poor sleep can have an impact on your health. It can lead to unwelcome sleepiness at inopportune moments, which can be potentially dangerous, cause accidents that are otherwise avoidable, and reduce productivity. You can lose the enjoyment of a good night's sleep and become more irritable and derive less enjoyment from life.

Your sleep

If you suffer from any of the following complaints you are likely to be suffering from a sleep problem or disorder and will benefit from following this course. Even if you do not, this course will help you to get the most out of your sleep.

You will benefit from this course if: -

- You are always tired
- You snore excessively
- You pause in your breathing as you sleep
- You have difficulty getting to sleep
- You can't stay asleep
- You fall asleep too easily
- You can't wake up in morning.

How to follow this course

As with the other courses within the *Oxford Centre for the Mind* series of courses, you need to approach this course from a practical point of view. You will not obtain the benefits that you can derive from this course unless you do the exercises that we outline and make the changes that we advise. Some of the changes that you decide to make may need the help of your partner. If this is the case, discuss the changes that you plan to make with them and ensure that you are both happy with your plans.

Before you start, it is important that you establish what your motivations are. To obtain the benefits that you can from this course, you need to follow through with the suggestions that we make, and to do so, you might wish to use the techniques outlined in our *Goals Course* and the *States of Mind Course* to achieve and maintain motivation.

We suggest that you brainstorm to identify the benefits that you could obtain from following this course. Take two minutes to do this now. Space is provided at page 55. At the same time, do all that you can to identify the ways in which your life until now has been limited by insufficient rest and excessive tiredness. As you work through the course, update your motivations. You may become aware of hidden benefits and motivations that you are not currently aware of.

It is important that you persevere with the changes that you decide to make in this course. Your aim should be to obtain good quality sleep by establishing good habits that you can live with throughout the rest of your life. Remember that any changes that you make may take up to three weeks before they have any noticeable effects.

How the course is structured

This course is divided into different sections. We suggest that you work through no more than one section per day and note any decisions that you make. Space is provided for this at page 56.

The changes that you make will usually take about three weeks to become established as habits. If you decide to adjust the rhythms of sleep and wakefulness, do not adjust your daily sleep and waking hours by more than one hour a day.

Measurement

You will be asked to do various assessments of your sleep in the section headed *'Assessing your sleep'* on page 22. Make sure to repeat these assessments at intervals of seven, fourteen and twenty-one days to see how the changes that you make are affecting your sleep. Repeat the tests and make the necessary adjustments, particularly to your preferred bedtime, as necessary.

Onword

In the next section we outline what sleep consists of and what happens while you are asleep, outlining different kinds of sleep and their functions. We will then identify a number of sleep disorders and outline the effects that these can have on your life. We will help you to assess whether you are experiencing difficulties with sleep or have a sleep disorder.

The sections after that will help you to improve your fitness for sleep and help to eliminate the elements that may cause you to experience poor quality sleep.

You will establish the amount of time that you need to obtain a good night's sleep and work out the best time for you to go to bed. We will provide various different strategies that you can use depending on what your daily schedule is.

After that we will outline what you can do to get to sleep at night, including how to reach the appropriate mental states that will help you to get to sleep easily and eliminate distracting worries, as well as outlining how you can use napping as a means of improving your quality of rest.

We will show you how to maximise the quality of your sleep by creating a good environment to sleep in, and show you how to change your lifestyle to optimise the quality of your sleep.

Finally, we comment briefly on how you can use sleep positively to enhance your life, discussing dreams, what they might mean and how they can be used to improve your enjoyment of life.

TWO

SLEEP OVERVIEW

In this section we discuss what sleep is, and what happens to the body and brain during a typical night's sleep. We explain how establishing a balance between sleep and wakefulness is important and discuss various problems that you might have with your sleep and help you to assess these problems.

What is sleep?

Sleep is a state in which we are disconnected from the outside world. We are unconscious of what is going on about us and we are generally unresponsive to external stimuli. We have no short-term memory and we generally do not connect with our five senses. Depending on the individual, the disconnection that we experience can be reversed either very easily or with great difficulty. Some people are easy to wake up, whereas others only wake up very slowly and remain groggy for a while. Generally, though, sleep is, and should be, easily reversible. It is possible to be in a deep sleep and yet within a few minutes be wide-awake.

Despite the fact that we are disconnected from the world during sleep, a number of activities are still ongoing within us. We continue to breathe, our hearts continue to beat, and a number of brain and mental functions continue to operate. For instance, our brains, cells and digestion can be as active as during the day.

Sleep is not the same as merely resting. Resting occurs during periods of wakefulness when the body is inactive and the mind is relaxed.

Functions of sleep

It is not clear exactly what the purpose of sleep is, however a number of changes take place during sleep and it may be that its purpose is to facilitate these changes.

Bodily and mental stress is reduced. Circuits within the brain have the opportunity to rest. Memories are consolidated and various other psychological changes occur. Sleep is necessary for these changes to happen properly. For instance, if students are deprived of sleep, their learning and memories will be hampered. This means that when studying for exams all-night cramming is actually detrimental to remembering whereas a good night's sleep will aid the forming of memories.

Is it possible to do without sleep?

It might seem that we could be much more productive and get much more done in our lives if we could eliminate the need to sleep. Many people have attempted to do this but no one has yet succeeded. In fact, the longest anybody has gone without sleep is about 260 hours. The absolute minimum amount of sleep that we are able to live on appears to be about four hours a night. If people get less sleep than this they feel unwell and excessively tired.

People who have been deprived of sleep for long periods of time can suffer from neurological symptoms, including paranoia and hallucinations. These symptoms are usually reversed as soon as the subject gets some sleep.

As far as we are aware, all animals sleep to a greater or lesser extent. This would appear bear out the fact that sleep is necessary for all living things, including humans.

The stages of sleep

Sleep does not consist of one continuous state. Instead, there are about four or five cycles of sleep during the night. These cycles last from about ninety minutes to two hours, with intervals of deep and light sleep and even wakefulness.

Each of these cycles has two separate phases.

Quiet sleep

The first phase is known as *quiet sleep*. During this phase the brain is at its most relaxed. The body is immobile, some digestion continues to occur and bodily repair is undertaken. The heart and breathing rate as well as blood pressure are at their lowest and because of this so is the level of stress on the heart. Brainwaves are large and slow at this time. If you wake up feeling tired and not fully refreshed it is likely to be because you were disturbed during quiet sleep.

Quiet sleep itself has three stages. The first stage is a transition into sleep during which consciousness is relinquished. For a person obtaining good quality sleep, this should only take a few minutes. The next stage, which may last up to half an hour, establishes a framework during which preparation is made for the third stage. This third stage is called *delta sleep*, and is the deepest form of sleep during the night. It consists of large, slow brainwave patterns. Young children experience a higher proportion of delta sleep – as much as a third of the time they spend asleep is delta sleep. This proportion falls as you get older: for the elderly it is as little as 10 per cent.

If you go a long time without sleep, you fall into quiet sleep very quickly and experience a longer phase of quiet sleep than you normally would.

R.E.M. sleep / paradoxical sleep

The second phase of sleep is known as *R.E.M. sleep* (*Rapid Eye Movement* sleep), also known as *paradoxical sleep*. This happens at the end of each of the sleep cycles and lasts for about thirty minutes. Episodes of R.E.M. sleep get longer and become closer nearer the end of night.

It is during R.E.M. sleep that dreaming occurs. To ensure that your dreams do not affect how your body behaves during sleep, hormones are released that paralyse your body, preventing you from injuring yourself as you act out dreams. At this time you lose the ability to control your bodily temperature and so both shivering and sweating cease. The muscles in your rib cage are paralysed, and so you need to breathe deeply through the diaphragm. Diaphragmatic breathing is generally positive because it draws more air into deep lobes of the lungs, but it can be problematical for obese people to breathe this way while they are in a prone position.

Waking phases

You will wake up during the night as many as seven times. However, it is unlikely that you will remember these periods of wakefulness. You will only remember them if you wake up for two minutes or more.

Establishing a balance between sleep and waking

The time that you spend asleep affects the quality of the time that you spend awake. Similarly, the time that you spend awake affects the quality of your sleep. So, you need to establish an optimal balance between sleep and wakefulness.

The longer that you spend awake, the more you will need to sleep and the more likely you will be to fall asleep. You will be accumulating a sleep debt that you will need to repay at some time. If you do lose sleep, you will need to catch up on your sleep, but you will not need to catch up on as much as you have lost. For instance, if you lose, say, three hours' sleep during one night, you will not need to get three hours' extra sleep over the following nights to catch up. This is because you sleep much more intensely during the start of a sleeping phase enabling greater recovery.

This balance between sleep and catch-up usually happens over a seven-day period, which ties in neatly with the seven days of the week. This means that you can catch up with any sleep you lose during the week at the weekend.

You also need to take into account your daily biological cycle (also known as your *circadian rhythms*). One of these rhythms concerns your body temperature. Your temperature varies during the day, responding to your energy requirements. It is highest around the middle of the day, dropping off throughout the afternoon, evening and night until it bottoms out about 3 am to 5 am, after which it starts rising again.

It is easier to fall asleep when the body temperature is falling – in the early afternoon and evening – and easier to wake up when the temperature is rising again in the morning.

Disrupting our sleep rhythms can also cause problems with our ability to sleep well. Many people find it difficult to get to sleep in the two hours before their normal bedtime. This is often noticeable on Sunday nights, when people go to bed early to get a good night's sleep in preparation for work the following day.

Having said that, you can, of course, adjust the amounts of sleep you need, within certain limits. You do not need exactly the same amount of sleep each night. If you are busy you can take a little less sleep during the week, but you will need to pay off this sleep debt at the weekend or by additional napping.

Identifying sleep problems

If you are to improve the quality of your sleep, you need to recognise that you may be suffering from a number of problems. Some of these you may be able to identify by yourself, for others you may need the help of someone else. These problems may vary from minor inconveniences, to major problems that can lead to illness and premature death. Some of these problems may arise due to the balance between sleep and wakefulness being disrupted.

Do you suffer from any of the following problems?

Insomnia

Insomnia is difficulty in falling asleep and affects about a third of us at some point. Insomnia can have a number of causes, including pain, stress, depression, anxiety and unhealthy living. Some insomnia may result from severe psychological trauma and as a result you may need psychological counselling to deal with it.

If you experience this disorder, you are likely to be sleepy a large proportion of the time and are likely to need an alarm clock to ensure that you wake up on time. You will probably need to sleep in and nap during the day or at weekends to catch up. You will feel better if you get more sleep.

Insufficient sleep disorder

This disorder is due to not obtaining enough sleep. It is often the case that most of us would benefit from more sleep. This does not necessarily mean spending more time in bed, though. It may be that you are spending a lot of time in bed but not getting good quality sleep. This course will help you to improve the quality of your sleep.

Breathing problems

Breathing problems during sleep affect about ten per cent of men and five per cent of women. This can range from light snoring to complete pauses in breathing, which can last from a few seconds to one or two minutes, and which may be repeated many times an hour.

If you have problems breathing during the night, this is likely to reduce the flow of oxygen going to the brain, potentially causing brain damage or mental problems. You are likely to be too sleepy when awake and have high blood pressure.

Sleepiness

Sleepiness is the feeling that you are tired and want to go to sleep, and you feel better when you get some sleep. It is possible to be sleepy without knowing it. This is especially the case if you are masking the symptoms of sleepiness with stimulants such as coffee.

If you suffer from excessive sleepiness you are liable to have impaired judgement and may nod off when carrying out various tasks and activities. This can be very dangerous if you are driving or performing similar tasks that require your full attention.

If you find yourself nodding off in such a situation, stop what you are doing and rest immediately (or as soon as it is safe to stop). If you haven't slept for a while, that is for more than a day, do not do anything that requires your full attention.

It has been estimated that the dangers associated with excessive sleepiness cause between thirty and fifty per cent of all accidents, and so if we could reduce the problems associated with excessive sleepiness, the world would be a safer place to live in.

Other health implications

Over a five to ten year period, sleep disorders raise the possibility of premature death. For example, breathing problems during sleep lead to raised blood pressure which can in turn lead to heart damage.

The digestive system can be adversely affected by poor sleep rhythms. Your digestive rhythms are not controlled simply by when you eat but also by your daily biological rhythms. If these rhythms are disrupted, digestive acid can be secreted at the wrong time causing damage to the inner lining of the gastro-intestinal tract.

Other problems associated with poor sleep are the loss of a restful night's sleep and consequent psychological problems – mood and quality of life are likely to be adversely affected over the long term, causing irritability and depression. Losing the restful effects of night's sleep lead may also lead to premature ageing.

Onword

You should now be familiar with the purpose, structure and rhythms of sleep and also with the some of the problems that people have with their sleep. In the following section, we will help you to assess the quality of your own sleep.

THREE

ASSESSING YOUR SLEEP

In this section we will give you the opportunity to assess your quality of your sleep and help to identify certain specific problems. The following sections will help you to deal with any problems that you might identify.

Assess your sleep

The following questions will help you to determine the quality of your sleep. Add up the number of positive answers that you give and highlight those which generally happen more than three times a week. Record your score on page 57.

1. Do you sleep for less than six hours in a twenty-four hour period?
2. Do you sleep for more than nine hours in a twenty-four hour period?
3. Do you get less sleep than you would like?
4. Do you find that your sleep is less refreshing than you would like it to be?
5. Do you take more than thirty minutes to get to sleep?
6. Are you awake for more than thirty minutes during the night?
7. Have you woken more than four times during the night, or during your main sleep period?
8. Do you need to go to the bathroom more than twice during the night?
9. Do you take more than twenty minutes to get back to sleep if you wake up?
10. Do you feel sleepy during the day?
11. Do you walk during your sleep?
12. Do you wake up with a gasp or a choke?
13. Do you find that your sleep is disturbed by pain or discomfort?

14. Is your sleep disturbed by noise, heat, light, your children, partner or your pets?

If you answered *no* to all of these questions you are getting good sleep. If you answered yes to any of them focus on these, particularly those you identified as occurring more than three times a week.

For example, if you find that you can fall asleep at any time, this is not a good sign, but a sign of poor health. Your goal should be to get to sleep within twenty minutes at bedtime. At other times during the day, you should find it difficult to get to sleep in less than thirty minutes.

The following two tests will help you to assess whether you are obtaining good quality sleep.

Assessing your sleepiness

These questions will help to assess your chances of dozing off. Ask yourself whether you can doze off in the following situations. If there is no chance, score zero. If there is a slight chance, score one. If there is a reasonable chance, score two and if there is a high chance score three. Record your score on page 58.

Do you doze while: -

1. Sitting and reading?
2. Watching television?
3. Sitting in the theatre, at meetings, at the cinema or in other similar environment?
4. Travelling as a passenger in a car for an hour?
5. Lying down to rest in the afternoon?
6. Sitting talking to someone?
7. Sitting quietly after lunch (not having drunk any alcohol)?
8. In a car that has stopped for a short while?

If your score is seven or less, you are able to benefit from this course. If your score is over twelve, then you should consult your doctor. If your score is between seven and twelve, then your actions should vary depending on the circumstances. In any case, this assessment will help you to become more aware of the state of your health and the state of your sleep.

Assessing the quality of your sleep

These questions will help you to assess the quality of your sleep.

If you answer no to all of the following questions, then you are getting sufficient good quality sleep for long-term health. If you answer yes to any questions you will benefit from this course. If you answer yes to three or more questions or yes to any of questions seven, eight, nine or eleven, then you should consult your doctor.

Note that these questions do not apply for the last thirty minutes before you go to sleep and the first fifteen minutes after you wake up.

Answer *yes* if any of the following have occurred at least three times a week over the last two months? Record your score on page 59.

1. Have you been sleepier than would have liked?
2. Have you taken any intentional or unintentional naps that have lasted for more than five minutes?
3. Have you slept for more than nine hours in a twenty-four hour period?
4. Have you been unable to stay awake during film that you were enjoying?
5. Have you deferred activities because you were too tired?
6. Have you fallen asleep without warning?
7. Have you tried actively to keep yourself awake?
8. Have you made mistakes because of sleepiness?
9. Have you struggled with sleepiness while performing a task or activity that required your full attention?
10. Have you had to stop doing something because of sleepiness or excessive fatigue?

11. Could you have fallen asleep within twenty minutes at anytime if you were comfortable, relaxed and undisturbed?

Do you suffer from any of the following problems?

Insomnia

You are likely to be suffering from insomnia if you take thirty minutes or more to get to sleep at the start of the night or similarly if you take that long to get back to sleep after you have woken up during the night. Also, if you are awake earlier than you would like to be, but cannot get back to sleep.

Insufficient sleep disorder

You may be suffering from this if you are always sleepy, if you need an alarm clock to wake up at weekends, if you need to take extra sleep to catch up at weekends or if you feel less sleepy when you manage to relax on your holidays because you have had the chance to catch up on your sleep.

Breathing problems - harmless snoring

If you snore loudly but are never sleepy and have never had any problems with your heart or blood pressure, than you have nothing to worry about here.

Breathing problems - sleep apnoea / upper airway resistance syndrome

If you stop breathing for short periods, if you snore loudly and wake up with a sudden burst, such as a gasp or cough, if you experience unwelcome sleepiness and heart problems or high blood pressure then you may have serious breathing problems. This course will help you to improve your sleep, but you should also consult your doctor.

Onword

In the following section, we will consider what you can do to eliminate a number of the problems relating to sleepiness and excessive tiredness by discussing the timing of your sleep and the time you spend in bed.

FOUR

TIMING YOUR SLEEP

The purpose of this section is to help you to establish your preferred amount of time in bed and to develop a bedtime regime that will enable you to get a good night's sleep.

Establishing the time you spend asleep

Over the next seven days make a note to add up all the time you spend asleep each day (not in bed, but actually asleep).

Include time you spend napping or dozing in front of the television. Include any extra hours you spend asleep at weekends. Do not include any time that you spend in bed awake. Record your daily totals on page 60.

When you have established this figure, divide the answer by seven. This will tell you how much sleep you need each night. Record this figure at page 60 under *figure A*, rounding it to the nearest fifteen minutes.

Establish your opportunity for sleep

Over the same seven-day period, calculate the amount of time that you have available to sleep. This will mainly be the time you spend in bed. Include the time that you spend in bed trying to go to sleep, but exclude any time that you are in bed doing something else, such as reading, listening to music, making love and so on.

Add on any time that you spend asleep or trying to get to sleep outside bed, such as time spent napping on a sofa in front of the television. Record your daily totals on page 60.

When you have established this figure, divide the answer by seven. This will tell you how much time you have available for sleep each day. Record this figure at page 60, under *figure B*, rounding it to the nearest fifteen minutes.

Your preferred time in bed

Now you will calculate your preferred time in bed, using the two figures that you have already calculated: that is, the *time you spend asleep* and your *opportunity for sleep*.

Record your preferred time in bed at page 60 under *figure C*.

To establish your preferred time in bed, decide which, if any, of the following categories you fall into.

Category 1

You are not sleepy when you are awake, but you have trouble getting to sleep at night – that is, you take more than thirty minutes to get to sleep.

If you fall into this category, add half an hour to the figure you arrived at when you calculated the time you spend asleep (*figure A*). For example, if you spend seven hours asleep, amend this figure to seven and a half hours. If the amended figure is still less than six hours, make it six hours.

Record this figure at page 60 under *figure C*.

Category 2

You are too sleepy when you are awake and have little trouble – that is, you spend less than thirty minutes - getting to sleep at night. If you fall into this category, add half an hour to the figure you calculated as your opportunity for sleep (*figure B*) to give your preferred time in bed.

Record this figure at page 60 under *figure C*.

Category 3

You are sleepy when you are awake and you have trouble getting to sleep at night. If you fall into this category, then add one hour to the time you calculated for the time you spend asleep (*figure A*) to establish your preferred time in bed (*figure C*). Record this figure at page 60.

Category 4

If none of the other categories apply, remain with your current sleeping pattern spending as much time asleep in bed as you do now. Record this figure at page 60.

Your aim

Aim to be in bed for the amount of time you calculated for your preferred time in bed (*figure C*). If this means spending more time in bed than you are at present, aim to go to bed earlier.

If you are tired but your preferred time in bed is a reduction on the amount of time than you are getting at present, you may be getting to much sleep, but poor quality sleep. Aim to improve the quality of your sleep.

Amending your calculations

Return to the calculations that you have made once a week over the next four weeks and reassess how you feel. Use this opportunity to make any necessary amendments to the figures you have reached. As you are now focused on your sleep, you will be becoming more aware of your needs and the figures you reached may need some adjustment.

Establishing your preferred bedtime

The aim of this section is to establish a regular bedtime that is right for you. Do this by working out your preferred *waking up time* and working backwards to calculate your bedtime: that is, the time you turn the lights out and start trying to go to sleep.

There are two keys to this. The first key is regularity. This will establish your sleeping cycle as part of a regular biochemical cycle. Even if your daily work / life schedule is erratic and irregular, aim to make your sleep periods as regular as you possibly can.

The second key is to establish a good bedtime regime. Your goal here is to establish a routine that readies you physically and mentally for sleep. To establish this you will need to establish a regime that you stick to for at least three weeks.

By preparing a routine that readies you for bed, you will already be prepared for the following day and your levels of anxiety will be reduced.

Decide which of the following categories you fall into:

Regular schedule

You fall into this category if you have a regular schedule, and you do not generally do any work between 7pm and 7am - this will be most people that have regular day jobs.

Decide on the time of day that you need to get up in order to get to work on time. Make a list of all the things that you need to do between getting up and starting work, including washing, eating breakfast, travelling and so on. Space is provided to do this at page 61. It may be that you are doing things in the morning that you can do better the night before (see below) meaning that you are having to get up earlier than necessary.

Once you have calculated the time that you need to get up, count back from this time the number of hours you found for your preferred time in bed (*Figure C* recorded at page 60). This is the time that you should be going to bed, turning the lights out and start going to sleep. Record this at page 61.

If you intend to use the bed for other reasons (such as reading, watching television, or making love) go to bed earlier. Maintain your aim to start going to sleep at the time you have already calculated.

Try to stick to this bedtime seven days a week if you can. It is best to do this, but you need not be completely inflexible. You can make your bedtime ninety minutes later or thirty minutes earlier at weekends if you want.

Early schedule

You fall into this category if you have to be at work before 7am. If this is the case, it is vital that you have you have a regular schedule.

Decide on the time of day that you need to get up in order to get to work on time. Make a list of all the things that you need to do between getting up and starting work, including washing, eating breakfast, travelling and so on. Space is provided to do this at page 61. It may be that you are doing things in the morning that you can do better the night before (see below) meaning that you are having to get up earlier than necessary.

Once you have calculated the time that you need to get up, count back from this time the number of hours you found for your preferred time in bed (*Figure C* recorded at page 60). This is the time that you should be going to bed, turning the lights out and start going to sleep. Record this at page 61.

Try to stick to this bedtime seven days a week if you can. It is best to do this, but you need not be completely inflexible. You can make your bedtime ninety minutes later or thirty minutes earlier at weekends if you want.

Late schedule

You fall into this category if you arrive home between 11pm and 3am.

If this is you, go to bed as soon as you get home and aim to be asleep within twenty minutes. If you find this difficult because you need to wind down, aim to be asleep within 30 to 60 minutes. Avoid having a big meal before you go to bed and avoid doing any more work.

Record your preferred time bedtime for work days on page 62. It doesn't matter what time you go to bed on your days off. Choose the times that are best for you.

Working nights

If you work nights, the most important thing is to go to sleep and have your main meal within a two to three hour period every day. This will help to anchor your sleep periods.

Unless you are able to sleep happily in one period, feel free to divide your sleep into two periods throughout the day. During your main sleep period, aim to get three or more hours sleep. Take a secondary sleep period between 2pm and 6 pm. Record your preferred primary and secondary sleep zones at page 62.

Take any naps you need to anticipate future sleepiness.

Variable and disrupted sleep patterns

If you have a variable work pattern, do whatever you can to achieve a constant pattern of sleep. Try to get three to four hours good sleep at the same time of day.

Prioritise sleep during the night and top up with naps, so that you never get sleepy. Get used to quality sleep in short periods of time.

Do whatever you can to stick to a routine. Prepare a day beforehand and video any television programmes that you want to watch so that you don't change your schedule for television.

Record your preferred sleep period at page 63.

If you live with other people in your house, and your sleeping pattern is such that you are asleep when others are awake, make sure that you have at least a four-hour period that is entirely for you to sleep in, during which no one is allowed to disturb you.

Preparing for bed

The purpose here is to prepare you for bed so that by the time you get to bed you have done everything you need to do and have left no outstanding tasks to worry about, ensuring that you can get to bed on time and in the right frame of mind.

Exercise

Over the next week, write down all of the things that you have to do before you go to bed. Write down the order that you do them and then schedule them so that you can get to bed on time. If you have some things that you have to do on certain days, such as weekends, make a separate list for that day. Space is provided for this on page 64.

Once you have done this, schedule each task. Work out how long each one takes to do and place them in the order that you normally do them.

Now be prepared to rearrange your schedule so that it helps you to get to sleep.

During the last two hours before you go to bed, avoid large meals and alcohol. Only eat easily digested foods like fruit. During this time, avoid doing any activity that will cause you stress, or excessive mental or physical effort. So avoid discussing family problems or matters such as finances. Avoid any exercise during this period.

If you can, avoid watching television in the last hour before you go to bed. You may try to stay up to see the end of a programme and then maybe go on to watch the next one, cutting into your sleep time. Also, certain television programmes might get your mind racing.

In the final half hour before you go to bed, do only relaxing activities.

Taking these factors into account, examine your pre-bed routine to see whether it needs amending. Do you need to consider taking meals earlier in the evening, for example?

If, having done this, you find that you are still having trouble getting to sleep, try incorporating a warm (but not hot) shower or bath into your routine. You stand a better chance of getting to sleep when your body temperature is falling, and taking a bath or shower will set you up for such a fall in temperature when you go to bed.

If you do have a shower or bath, make sure that it is not too hot, as this will raise your body temperature excessively. Remember to amend your pre-bed schedule accordingly.

In bed

When you go to bed, avoid going to sleep with the television, radio or lights on (dim lighting is okay but avoid bright lights). These are all stimulants and will deprive you of good quality sleep.

Onword

Having determined the amount of time you need to spend in bed and established your preferred bedtime and pre-bed routine, in the following section, we look at how you can get to sleep if you are having difficulties, deal with sleepiness and use napping to improve the quality of your days and nights.

FIVE

SLEEPING

In this section we deal with the actual business of sleeping. Firstly we look at how you can go about getting to sleep. If you have problems getting to sleep, regularly taking at least thirty minutes, then this section may help you. We also outline how you can use naps to you avoid sleepiness and thus feel fully alert throughout the waking periods of your day. Finally, we look at other strategies to avoid sleepiness.

Getting to sleep

Most people experience trouble getting to sleep at some point during their lives. Getting to sleep easily is a question of mental focus - that is, ensuring that your mind is in the right state of mind for getting to sleep easily. Make your aim to associate being in bed with getting to sleep, not with worrying about getting to sleep.

Problems getting to sleep

Often when we are lying in bed, with nothing to do, the mind can start focusing on worrying matters. Your brain might start racing, and if you are in a particular frame of mind, such as being angry or frustrated, you are likely to have difficulty switching off. Then when sleep fails to come, the level of frustration increases making it even less likely.

Strategies to get to sleep

One problem with being in the right state of mind to get to sleep is that *trying* to get to sleep is the worst thing you can do. Trying is associated with mental effort and sleep is associated with a letting go of mental effort.

Firstly, if you have a clock that you can see during the night, turn it away from you so that you cannot see it. Watching time drag by can only increase your frustration.

If you find that your mind has a tendency to race as you are going to sleep, there are a number of things that you can do. Make a note of the things that you tend to think about. Record these thoughts at page 65. When you have done so, look at what you have written, either during the night or the following day.

If you have identified certain anxieties, the best approach to take is to do all that you can to deal with the causes of your anxiety before you go to bed. This may mean doing something in the evening or even during the day beforehand. Is the anxiety caused by home life? Work life? Both? Or something else? You will find that it is always better to deal with causes of anxiety than to put them off. In the *Concentration & Focus* course we explain that our troubles are very rarely rooted in the present, but are usually rooted in something that has happened in the past, or to do with worries about what will happen in the future. In the *States of Mind* course, we outline various strategies for dealing with these concerns. The strategies outline in these two courses will help you to deal with any anxieties you feel.

If you have not been able to deal with your problems during the day, decide on a procedure that will help you to deal with them whenever you can. You will find it easier if you prepare your strategy out of bed with the lights on. Set aside between ten minutes to half an hour to really think about the problem and work out how you are going to deal with it. Write down your thoughts. This will help you to become clearer about them. Space is provided at page 66.

Be as honest with yourself as you can be. Ask yourself how the problem is bothering you. Ask yourself what would happen if the worst possible consequence happens. If you do find yourself dwelling on these thoughts again during the night, feel free to return to your written notes. Consult them as many times as necessary. This will help you to deal with the source of your anxiety and get to the root of the problem all the more quickly.

Feel free to refer to courses on *Goals* and *States of Mind* as well and use the strategies we outline there. Remember that in the *Goals* course we said that what ultimately motivates us is the pursuit of pleasure or the avoidance of pain. The exercises in those courses will help you to deal with the causes of your anxiety and find strategies that will give you a way out.

Additionally, you can make use of the concentration exercises outlined in the *Concentration & Focus* course, when you are actually lying down and going to sleep. These exercises are designed to slow your breathing and metabolism, and still your mind. Thus, they are ideal for putting you into a state of mind conducive to sleep.

If you find that your mind is still racing, try using relaxation tapes, or tapes that play relaxing instrumental music. If you can, ensure that the tape switches itself off automatically when it is finished. This will mean that it doesn't affect you while you are asleep. Avoid listening to the radio though as any speech is likely to be distracting.

Dealing with physical anxiety

Another possible cause of trouble getting to sleep may be physical tension. If this is so there are various exercises courses you can do that are designed to eliminate excessive tension from your body, such as yoga or pilates.

If, having followed these suggestions your mind is still racing, it might be that the problem you are suffering from is more serious, and you may need to consult your doctor. For instance, consult your doctor if you are suffering from a racing heart, panic attacks, feelings of hopelessness, or if you feel suicidal.

If sleep is not imminent

If you think that you are not likely to get to sleep within the next thirty minutes when your go to bed, or within ten minutes during the night, and if sleep is getting less, not more, likely, get out of bed. This way you will avoid associating bed with problems getting to sleep.

Once you are out of bed, make sure that you keep warm and comfortable. Do only relaxing activities such as reading a book or taking a bath. Drink a warm caffeine free drink, such as warm milk. Avoid drinking anything with caffeine in it such as coffee or tea. Don't watch television, as it can be easy to get drawn into whatever is showing

Return to bed when you start to feel sleepy, but don't expect to fall asleep straight away. This expectation is likely to put added pressure on you to get back to sleep. Just relax and allow sleep to come.

Napping

A nap is a short period of sleep outside your main sleep period. A nap can be either positive or negative. A positive nap will be enjoyable, refreshing and make you feel more alert. A negative nap will make you feel groggy and may prevent you from sleeping in your main sleep period.

When should you nap?

You should certainly nap when you are dangerously sleepy: that is, when you find your head nodding, when you have an irresistible urge to sleep, when your eyes are closing or when you cannot focus your mind. If these symptoms are not remedied by becoming physically active take a nap.

If you have a regular daily schedule, you should only have to nap rarely and you should know the reason why you need to nap. For instance, if your daily schedule has been disturbed for some reason.

If you do not have a regular schedule then take naps when you need them. You could even make extended naps a regular thing and make them part of your sleep schedule.

Power napping

Power napping is useful if your sleep is constrained by a busy schedule. For example, if you have a very busy work schedule or if you have a small child or baby.

The duration of these naps is a matter of choice, but should be between ten and twenty-five minutes. It is more important to be quiet and relax fully than actually to fall sleep. If you adopt the mental approach outlined in the *Concentration & Focus* course, you should be fine.

Dealing with sleepiness

If you can fall asleep at any time, this is not a sign of good health. You may be suffering from excessive sleepiness. You should ideally feel sleepy just before you go to sleep and just after you wake up.

Sleepiness is caused either by failing to get enough sleep or by getting too much poor quality sleep. The strategies outlined in the rest of this course will help you to deal with most of the causes of unwelcome sleepiness. However, you also need to know what to do if you feel sleepy in the short term.

Whenever you feel sleepy, make sure that you do not do anything that puts either yourself or other people at risk.

If unwelcome sleepiness is just coming on, do whatever you can to become more alert: get physically active and seek out light. Eat some food or drink coffee (usually we would suggest that you avoid coffee, but using it in situations like these will usually reduce sleepiness). Remember though that a stimulant like coffee will merely mask the symptoms of sleepiness. It will not deal with the underlying cause. Stimulate your mind by initiating a mental activity that will stop you from being bored.

If on the other hand, you are not busy, you could take a refreshing nap.

If you feel irresistibly sleepy (your head is starting to nod and you are struggling to keep your eyes open) during periods when you would expect to be awake, consider this an emergency situation. Stop whatever you are doing as soon as it is safe and rest.

You assessed whether you were excessively sleepy in the exercise on page 23. If you think that you may have a problem with sleepiness, keep a record of how your feel over a seven-day period, recording instances of sleepiness. Space is provided for this at page 67.

Highlight any dangerous or potentially dangerous situations. Learn to recognise the symptoms of sleepiness so that you can take pre-emptive action to deal with them before they become a problem.

If having made the changes recommended in this course, you still have a problem with excessive sleepiness, consult with your doctor.

Onword

The following section deals with various factors that may affect the quality of your sleep, and what you can do to ensure that you obtain good quality sleep.

SIX

QUALITY OF SLEEP

This section focuses on how you can improve the quality of your sleep. We examine how you can improve the environment you sleep in, including making your bedroom a place more amenable to sleep, using light and sound creatively, establishing the correct temperature to sleep well and ensuring that you bed is going to help you to get a good night's sleep. Go through each item and identify any changes that you are going to make. Record these on page 68.

Your sleeping environment

The bedroom

Your bedroom should ideally be reserved for sleep, making love, reading and dressing. Remove anything that is likely to induce stress or cause a stressful environment. For instance, do not turn your bedroom into an office, do not store documents in it. Keep all non-essential electrical equipment to a minimum. Remove computers, desks, work, filing cabinets and so on. Remove your television from your bedroom. A radio is okay, but avoid falling asleep with the radio on.

By making your bedroom an environment solely for sleeping in and keeping it free of work associations or other associations that might induce stress you will anchor your bedroom as a room associated with sleeping. This will help create the right environment for sleep. For more on anchors see our *States of Mind* course.

Temperature

The ambient temperature that is most likely to ensure sleep is about 16°C (65°F), which is a little cooler than the average household temperature. If you are able to adjust the temperature in your bedroom do so. You may be able to cool it down by leaving a window open, having a fan on or adjusting the air conditioning.

Noise

Noise can be a problem both when trying to get to sleep and during sleep. Excessive background noise may prevent you from getting to sleep but often it is the contrast between foreground and background noise that causes problems and not the level of noise itself. For instance, people who live near roads soon become accustomed to the incessant background noise of cars and generally do not have excessive difficulty getting to sleep.

Do your best to eliminate as much noise as you can when going to sleep. If you cannot, then you could try masking any leftover noise by using, say, a fan, or a white noise generator. White noise is the hiss that you get from an untuned radio or television. At low levels it can mask other noises without being distracting itself.

You could also try using earplugs, but make sure that you buy a good set and that you do not put them too deep in your ears, as they may become lodged there permanently

Light

Ensure that the lighting you have in your bedroom is appropriate for a bedroom environment: soothing, comfortable and not too bright.

When going to sleep, eliminate as much light as you can. Most people sleep better in complete darkness. If you fall into this category, do your best to ensure that your bedroom is completely dark when going to sleep. Consider installing shutters or blackout blinds.

If you find it difficult to get to sleep in complete darkness, consider installing a light with a very low wattage bulb. This will provide sufficient light to see by but will not be distracting with your eyes shut.

Light and your daily rhythms

We all have natural biochemical rhythms. These regulate, among other things, hormone production, eating and sleep. For some reason that no one yet knows, these daily rhythms run naturally on a 25, not 24-hour cycle, which means that without any other stimulation, you would tend to get up later and later in the day. In order to combat this, these rhythms are reset each day by exposure to daylight. Exposure to daylight will kick-start you into the day, just as removal of daylight starts off the processes that lead to you feeling tired and wanting to go to bed.

Knowing this, you can use light to improve the quality of your sleep (natural daylight is preferable to artificial light, even if it is cloudy).

If you sleep to a regular rhythm, ensure that you are exposed to light as you are waking up. This will help the process of waking up, making you feel more alert.

If your schedule is such that you have to wake up early, make sure that you are exposed to light in morning and avoid natural light in the evening.

If you wake up earlier than you would like to, expose yourself to light late in the afternoon, and avoid any exposure in the two hours after you wake up.

If you work a night shift, avoid bright light as much as you can after you have finished your shift. If it is safe to do so, try using dark glasses.

Be aware that for exposure to light to have an effect, it must be for a minimum of thirty minutes.

Your mattress

The mattress you sleep on is very important. Not only will it impact on the quality of your sleep, it will affect your body as a whole throughout your life. Remember that you spend approximately one third of your life in bed. If the mattress that you sleep on is poor, it will affect your postural muscles, particularly the muscles of the back, leading to the problems associated with poor posture. Shop around for a good mattress and do not skimp. That would be a false economy. Make sure that you have one that is firm and comfortable. Try sleeping in different beds until you find a mattress that is comfortable for you.

Turn your mattress regularly and replace it if it is older than twelve years old.

Pillows

Your pillows should be such that they do not induce any breathing problems. Your aim should be to keep your spine straight when you are sleeping. If you are sleeping in your side, ensure that your head is not drooping or propped up too much. Try to ensure that your back, throat and head are roughly in a straight line.

Onword

In this section we have looked at what you can do to improve the quality of your sleep. In the following one, we will consider this further by looking at what changes to your lifestyle might lead to an improvement in your sleep.

SEVEN

LIFESTYLE CONSIDERATIONS

In this section, we examine a number of changes you might want to consider making to your lifestyle that will help you to sleep better. As we have already said the quality of your waking life is dependent on the quality of your sleep, and the quality of your sleep is dependent on your waking life, so it is important to take care of the rest of your life.

There are, of course, a whole host of things that will affect the quality of your sleep. Many of our other courses will have a positive impact on your quality of life as a whole and accordingly on the quality of your sleep. You might particularly want to consider the following factors.

Physical exercise

If you do exercise of any sort, this will have a positive impact on your ability to sleep. The physical tiredness induced by cardiovascular exercise will ensure that your body is *properly* tired at the end of the day and ensure that you need sleep, helping to bring it on.

Flexibility exercises will ensure that your muscles are healthy, flexible and free of tension. This will help to prevent any niggles distracting you while you are going to sleep.

Even if you are not following a planned exercise regime, try and get half an hour's exercise or physical activity of some sort during the day. This could be something as mundane as walking or gardening.

Mental development

Our courses are all designed to help you master your mind. As you work through those courses, you will find yourself taking charge of your mind. You will be less prone to distraction and anxiety and more able to ensure the outcomes you want for yourself, including a good healthy night's sleep.

Healthy living

What, how and when you eat will affect the quality of your sleep. In our *Healthy Eating* course we suggest that avoiding non-fruit foods within two hours of going to bed will help to improve your digestion. Ensuring that your body is not engaged in energy-consuming digestion will also help you to get to sleep more easily.

Avoid stimulating drinks such as tea, coffee, and carbonated soda drinks containing sugar. Drinking these will not help you in getting to sleep. Also eliminate cigarettes, and recreational drugs and minimise your intake of alcohol.

Coffee

We all associate coffee with staying awake. It is the drink that we use to keep us running when we are tired. However, it is a chemical stimulant that can disrupt the efficient running of your body. The caffeine in coffee will only mask your sleepiness. The underlying causes will still be present, and so you are better off dealing with these. By adopting healthy eating and healthy sleeping strategies, you will ensure that your energy and alertness are maximised over the whole day, without any of the compensating energy slumps that you will get through consuming stimulants.

Overuse of coffee can actually reduce its effectiveness as a stimulant. It can disrupt your biochemical rhythms, actually causing you to feel sleepier at other periods in the day. It can also increase anxiety and tension.

To use coffee effectively as a stimulant, drink it in moderate amounts in one go, early on in the day. Drink no more than one cup per day.

If you are using coffee as an emergency stimulant to combat tiredness - when driving for example, remember that it will take twenty minutes to have an effect, and so refrain from any activity during that period, until you begin to feel more alert.

Artificial aids to sleep

Many people take sleeping drugs or alcohol to help them to get to sleep, believing that they cannot do so in any other way. It is generally not the case that we need artificial help getting to sleep. We have been designed by evolution to require sleep and all of us will eventually be able to get to sleep without any help. Drugs and alcohol are not a long-term cure and they may cause *rebound insomnia*, which can ultimately make your problems worse.

If you find that you need sleeping pills or alcohol to get to sleep then you are dealing with the symptoms of the problem and not the underlying cause. It is much better to find what is preventing you from getting to sleep in the first place and deal with that instead. If you are taking prescription drugs, however, do not stop taking them without first consulting your doctor. Doing so could be potentially hazardous.

Rebalancing your life

One other thing you could do is examine your life as a whole to see whether there is anything that you can change that will improve the quality of your life.

Find some activity that you can do that is fun, that is just for you, and which brings you pleasure. Also, find an activity that is altruistic, such as a charitable activity which improves the life of others. Either of these alternatives will help to improve the quality of your life, giving it a greater purpose. The benefits of doing so will permeate through your whole life, including your sleeping life.

Use the space provided on page 69 to identify at least five things that you could do which would make a difference to your lifestyle, and then go and do them. See whether they make a difference to the quality of your sleep over the next two weeks.

Your partner

It is usually the case that people who sleep together sleep better. However, this is not always so. Sometimes sleeping with a partner can be a liability. For instance, they might snore excessively or wake up and disturb you during the night. They may have a different work regime to you that means that they are getting up when you are trying to get to sleep.

If you have problems in this area, discuss them with your partner. Attempt to find a solution that benefits both of you. Initially, you might simply have to inform them that you are trying to improve the quality of your sleep and what your new requirements are. Attempt to find solutions that are mutually acceptable.

Make your search for a solution a positive one. Always look for solutions and focus on the problem not the person. For instance, if your partner's snoring is preventing you from getting to sleep, do not use this as a means of criticising them.

Ask yourself do you sleep better with or without your partner? Do you sleep better at home or away from home? Would you benefit from some form of background noise, such as a fan or white noise generator? Or earplugs? How would these affect your partner?

You may not always be able to negotiate everything that you want, so in some cases, sleeping in different rooms may be an answer. If so, consider whether it needs to be every day, or are you able to make alternative arrangements and sleep together, say, at weekends.

Reach a strategy that you can both agree on and stick with it. After a suitable amount of time review your strategy and see if you need to make any changes. Be sure not to allow the search for a solution to your sleeping difficulties to become a problem with your relationship as a whole.

Remember that if you can both get a good night's sleep, your lifestyle, health and mood will all benefit. So, then, in the long term, will your relationship with your partner.

Other night time disturbances

In addition to your partner there are a number of other potential causes of sleep disturbance. Three of these are your children, your pets and the phone.

Children

Unless you have a very young child, do your best to ensure that you are not disturbed more than once each night, as this will adversely affect your sleeping patterns.

Pets

The same applies to pets. Sleeping with a pet in your room is okay as long as it doesn't disturb you more than once per night. If it does, consider keeping your pet in another room during the night.

Phone

Unless you are in a job that requires you to be immediately contactable, such as an on-call doctor, make sure that the phone will not disturb you during the night. Ensure that you control the phone, do not let it control you. Most of the problems that are likely to come at you via the phone can wait until morning.

Problems with children, pets and the phone can be exacerbated if you are a shift worker, or sleep when others in the house are awake. Make it a rule that you have at least a four-hour period where you can sleep and during which no one else is allowed to disturb you.

Record any decisions you make concerning the factors raised in this section in your decisions section on page 69.

Onword

This concludes the sections of the course that deal with problems associated with sleeping and how to deal with them, by improving the timing and the quality of your sleep. The following section deals with how you can use sleep positively and creatively to enhance other areas of your life.

EIGHT

POWER SLEEP

Most of this course is concerned with eliminating problems with sleep, improving the timing of your sleep and doing what you can to improve the quality of your sleep. You can also make use of what you know about sleep to improve your performance during the day.

Upcoming events

If we have something important coming up, such as a speech or presentation, it can be the case that we might be tempted to change our regime. We all have the image of the genius who can work all night without needing sleep and who goes on to function brilliantly the following day. In fact, the truth is that we function better if we sleep properly.

If you do have an event in the near future in which you need to perform at your best, you need to prepare for it, and this includes focusing on your sleep. Remember that if you lose, say four hours' sleep because you are preparing for an upcoming event, you may have lost ten per cent of your sleep, which can be destabilising to your daily rhythms making you tired and lethargic during the day.

The best thing that you can do then, is to ensure that you are properly rested. Make sure that you stick to your sleep routine. Do whatever work you need to do during the day and then when you have finished, ensure that you wind down properly and get a good night's sleep. Have a notepad handy during the night so that you can record any extra thoughts that come to you. You will then be able to record your thoughts and let them go until morning, ensuring that you are properly refreshed.

Changing time zones

When you are travelling through different time zones, it is important to maintain all of your healthy living practices. You will be better prepared for a change in time zones if you are fit healthy, eating healthily and properly rested.

One thing you can to do to make sleep easier is to start to adjust your sleep times before you travel. If you will be going to bed earlier after you have travelled, start napping at your future bedtime before you travel. If you will be going to bed later after you travel, gradually delay your sleeping times, but ensure that you are still getting good quality sleep.

You can also manipulate your exposure to light to help to adjust your circadian rhythms.

Dreams

Recent research would seem to indicate that we dream throughout the time that we are asleep, but that the majority of dreaming takes place during R.E.M sleep.

We all dream, although we do not all remember our dreams. There are many superstitions associated with dreams. Some people believe that they can be used to predict the future. Others believe that if they die in their dreams they will die in real life.

In fact, little is known about dreams and why we dream. One theory is that we sleep in order to dream. Dreaming may be a way of processing the events that have happened to us during the day and making mental connections with other events in our lives. Our minds would need to do this during some sort of *downtime* during which no new sensory information is being processed. This may also explain why we often have dreams that seem bizarre and strange. Ours brains may simply be making subtle connections between two very different events. Since our memories are also based on making associations between different events and ideas, there may be a connection between our dreams and memory formation.

Dream diaries

You can enhance your dreams by making a decision to keep a dream diary. Write down whatever dreams you can remember as soon as you wake up. Not only will this help you to remember them, it might bring out the connections between different events in your life that you had not previously been aware of.

Do not simply record your dreams. Also record any thoughts that you have that accompany them. Ask yourself what your dreams might mean and record your answer. When you have done that, ask yourself why you answered that way. Doing this may help you to discover your deep motivations and learn more about yourself.

Onword

Having read through the course, you should now have all the information you need to ensure that you can obtain good quality sleep throughout your life.

Make sure that you commit to maintaining your new habits for the long term. Our *Goals* course will help any changes you make as a result of this course into changes that you incorporate into your life forever.

NINE

ENDWORD

You have now completed the *Sleep Course* and you should now have all the necessary skills and knowledge to ensure that you can get good quality sleep. Putting this knowledge to good use will help to ensure that you can perform optimally in all areas of your life.

TEN

MATERIALS

Exercise to identify the benefits of good sleep

Identify the benefits that could accrue to you by obtaining good quality sleep. Update this as you go through the course.

Identify any problems that you have that you could eliminate by getting good sleep.

Exercise to identify decisions that you make

Write down any decisions that you make, including changes to your sleep patterns, the time you go to bed, and anything you are going to do to improve the quality of your sleep. Also, identify any bad habits that you want to eliminate.

Assessing your sleep

Record your score here:

Record any yes answers that happen more than three times a week here:

Assessing your sleepiness

Record your score here:

Record any yes answers that happen more than three times a week here:

Assessing the quality of your sleep

Record your score here (remember only answer yes if occurrences happened more than three times during the last two months):

Establishing the time you spend asleep

Record the amount of time you spend asleep during a week here:

Divide this figure by seven to get a daily figure.
Record it here under Figure A. Remember to round to the nearest fifteen minutes.

Figure A:

Your opportunity for sleep

Record the amount of time you have available for sleep during the week here:

Divide this figure by seven to get a daily figure.
Record it here under Figure B. Remember to round to the nearest fifteen minutes.

Figure B:

Your preferred time in bed

Record which category you fall into here.

Calculate the amount of time you should be spending in bed and record it here under Figure C.

Figure C:

Pre-work routine

Make a list of the things that you need to do between getting up and getting to work here. Put them in order and decide how long each one takes to do:

Now go through your list and see if there is anything that you can eliminate from this list by moving it to the previous night. If so, record this on page 64, where you will record your pre-bed schedule.

Having trimmed your list, work back from the time you have to get to work, and work out what time you need to get out of bed. Record this time below.

Time to get out of bed:

Calculating your bed time

Deduct the figure you arrived at for your preferred time in bed (Figure C calculated at page 60)

Record your bedtime here. This is the time you will turn out the lights and start going to sleep.

Your lights out time:

Lights out time for those on a late schedule

Record your preferred lights out time here

Your lights out time:

Sleep periods for those working nights

Record your preferred lights out for your primary sleep period time here

Your main lights out time:

Record your preferred lights out time for your secondary sleep period here

Your secondary lights out time:

Sleep periods for variable and disrupted sleep patterns

Record your preferred sleep period here

Your lights out time:

Pre-bed routine

Make a list of the things that you need to do before you go to bed. Put them in order and decide how long each one takes to do:

Now schedule each task, recording how long each one takes and put them in the order you do them.

Make any necessary amendments to your schedule here

Difficulties with getting to sleep

Record any thoughts that you have when you are trying to get to sleep here (copy this page if necessary).

Strategies for dealing with anxiety

Decide what you are going to do to deal with your night-time anxieties and record you decisions here.

Record your sleepiness

Note down any instances of unwelcome sleepiness here.

Quality of sleep

Record any changes that you intend to make concerning the quality of sleep here.

Lifestyle changes

List five things you could do to make the quality of your life better.

Record any other changes that you intend to make concerning your lifestyle here.

More Quick Courses Coming Soon!

Visualisation

Analytical Thinking

Creative Thinking

Setting and Achieving Goals

Powerful States of Mind

Essential Communication Skills

Emulating Success

Healthy Eating

Healthy Sleep

4753361R00043

Printed in Germany
by Amazon Distribution
GmbH, Leipzig